I0447215

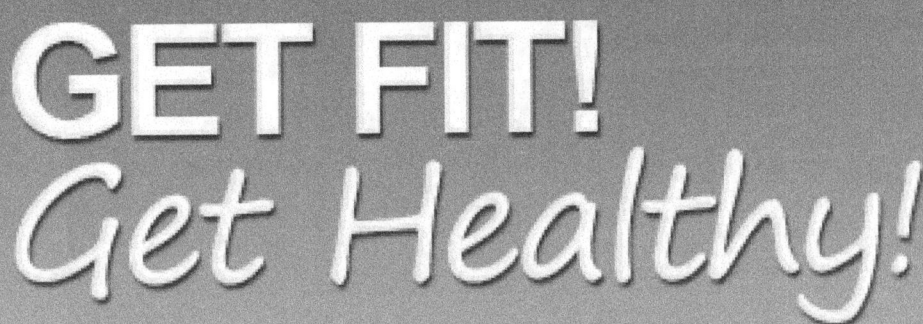

GET FIT!
Get Healthy!

101 Powerful Tips
For A Fitter, Healthier You!

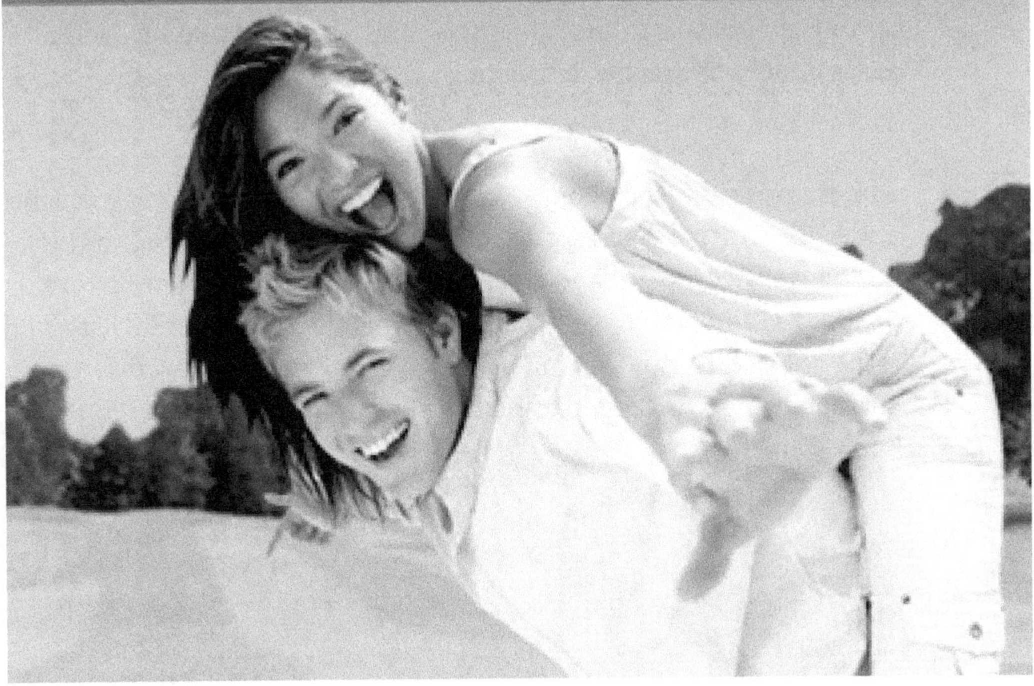

Disclaimer

This e-book has been written to provide information about Internet marketing. Every effort has been made to make this ebook as complete and accurate as possible. However, there may be mistakes in typography or content. Also, this e-book provides information only up to the publishing date. Therefore, this ebook should be used as a guide - not as the ultimate source.

The purpose of this ebook is to educate. The author and the publisher does not warrant that the information contained in this e-book is fully complete and shall not be responsible for any errors or omissions. The author and publisher shall have neither liability nor responsibility to any person or entity with respect to any loss or damage caused or alleged to be caused directly or indirectly by this e-book.

Table of Contents

Introduction

Fact: If you want more out of life, you need to be ready to commit more and invest more into staying fit and eating right.

While there have been innumerable diet plans and exercise programs sprouting like mushrooms nowadays -- all claiming to provide the fastest results – we all know the basic equation to staying fit and healthy is regular exercise and proper diet.

It has been called by many names, defined in so many ways and presented in so many forms but all health and fitness programs boils down to these two: DIET and EXERCISE. There is no other way to go about it – not, if you want lasting results.

And yet, despite this common knowledge on what needs to be done to stay fit and healthy, most of us struggle not to fall off the wagon, and many still have to contend with the frustrating battle of beating the bulge.

The weight loss industry has become a highly lucrative market, with food manufacturers, nutrition experts, and plastic surgeons all feeding from the growing desperation and depression of overweight and obesity.

But while the equation to fitness and health is so simple and straightforward, it remains a great challenge. With the demands of daily living – work-related stresses, social pressures, life changes, holidays, travels, winter seasons, and everything else in between – are all contributing factors that can disrupt fitness routines and upset diet regimens.

The real challenge here is on how you can possibly stay resolute and consistent with the program despite internal and external factors that often come into play.

This eBook is designed to help you equip yourself with tips, tricks and practical advice on how you can stay fit and healthy in the modern times.

It doesn't have to be a constant struggle. Fitness and healthy living is not a temporary phase or a convenient solution you can readily pull out from your closet in time for the summer season or during special occasions. If you want lasting results, ditch the 2-week plan or the 6-month program. Make health and fitness an integral part of your lifestyle, as it should be.

Read on and find out you can live, breath, eat, move and think healthy.

1   Stay hydrated.

This is one of the most important advices you can ever get when it comes to staying healthy and fit. Drinking water every chance you get, or at least every couple of hours. Water helps ensure your body systems will keep running smoothly and it also plays a vital role in weight loss. So don't forget to drink up.

2   Your mom was right, never skip breakfast.

You have probably heard it over and over how breakfast is the most important meal of the deal. And it really is. A lot of people seem to think skipping breakfast will help them lose weight faster. This could not be farther than the truth! According to numerous medical studies, people who skip this meal actually have increased risks of gaining weight.

Breakfast helps stabilize the body's metabolism. Ditching your first meal of the day will result to an increase in LDL levels or bad cholesterol and lower insulin levels. The increase in bad cholesterol in the body will result to clogged arteries, which can lead to a number of serious health complications such as heart disease. There is also that little known fact that people tend to take in higher calories all throughout the day after missing their breakfast. If you are trying to lose weight, have a small fruit, granola or yoghurt for breakfast.

3   Take fish oil supplements.

Recent studies conducted by University of Western Ontario revealed that regular intake of fish oil supplements can speed up burning of calories by as much as 400 more calories. Fish oil supplements are rich in Omega 3, which is also effective in the prevention of the hardening of the arteries, which is one of the leading causes of heart diseases. However, it is generally best to check with your physician first before adding fish oil supplements into your daily regimen.

4   Work up a sweat.

Make exercise a part of your daily routine. Regular exercise helps keep the heart healthy. There are number of ways you can incorporate exercise into your lifestyle, it's a matter of finding one that best suits you. Try to exercise at least 3 to 4 times a week, you will be surprised how much calories a simple jog or brisk walk can burn. To give you an idea, here are some few examples:

- Biking at a leisurely pace for 1 hour -- a total of 230 to 340 calories burned
- Walking at a moderate pace for 1 hour – a total of 205 to 300 calories burned

- Mowing the lawn for 1 hour – a total of 300 to 450 calories burned
- Jogging at a moderate pace for 1 hour -- a total of 300 to 600 calories burned

5   Add variety to your exercise routine.

Keep things light and fun by changing your fitness routine every now and then. Explore activities that aid weight loss, go outside and job along the park or by the beach. Consider taking up strength training, mountain climbing, cycling and other fun activities that can make exercise more fun and exciting.

6   Get enough sleep.

With the fast-paced lifestyle and grueling schedules, sleep is often taken for granted. An average person needs to have 7 to 8 hours of sleep every night. If you want to maintain a healthy weight, sleep should be given equal importance, as it is the only time the body can heal and repair itself. Lack of sleep also impairs brain function so make sure you get enough zzzzs.

7   Enjoy mind and body exercises.

Consider taking yoga or tai chi classes. These exercises do not only stretch your muscles as well as strengthen the bones, sinews and joints, it can also help you relax mentally.

Mind and body exercises are great way to wind down after a long and grueling day at work. It can help ease anxiety and pain as well as sped up recovery time.

8   Learn relaxation techniques.

It's no secret that stress can contribute to weight gain and development of chronic diseases. By learning relaxation responses, you can stop the adverse effects that come with stress. Among the popular relaxation techniques include breathing exercises, journaling, visualization and laughter, among others. If you deal with serious amount of stress on a daily basis, teach your body how to best cope with it.

9   Ditch the chips for healthier snack options.

Cultivate smarter food choices to stay fit and healthy. This includes choosing your snacks with more thought and consideration. If you enjoy a bag of chips while watching TV or movie, replace it healthier snack choices like a piece of apple, small yoghurt or whole wheat pita bread – all of which can satisfy your cravings minus the calories.

Keep your healthy snacks readily on hand so you won't be tempted to indulge in junk food. Make sure you don't have junk food and unhealthy food products on your desk and pantry. By keeping it out of sight, you won't feel deprived.

10   Discover the healthy goodness of green tea.

Take cure from the Japanese and discover how green tea can aid in rapid weight loss. You can use it to quench your thirst instead of soda and other fizzy drinks. Green tea have been known to work well with a number of health conditions include rheumatoid arthritis, cardiovascular diseases, impaired immune function, infections, high cholesterol levels and even certain forms of cancer.

11 Take vitamin supplements.

If you are trying to cut down on your calorie intake, chances are, you may be also compromising your nutrition. The best way to augment the depleted vitamins and minerals in the body is through supplementations. Discuss this with your physician and determine which type of supplementation will best address you nutrition requirements.

12 Wash your hands often.

One preventive measure to avoid getting sick or contamination is by washing hands thoroughly and regularly. This may be a very basic habit that has been inculcated in us since early childhood, but one that is sorely overlooked. Here are some guidelines on washing hands:

Wash hands before:

- Preparing meals
- Before eating
- Treating wounds
- Giving medication
- Caring for the injured and sick

Wash hands after:

- Handling food, especially when handling raw meat and poultry
- Using the toilet
- Changing diapers
- Touching toys, pets and waste

- Coughing, blowing of nose, and sneezing into hands
- Treating wounds
- Caring for the injured and sick
- Handling chemicals and garbage or anything that might be contaminated

13   Get rid of unhealthy vices.

Cultivate healthy habits and ditch the ones that pose adverse effects on your health. Anything in excess can be bad and you don't want your health to suffer the consequences.

14   Take annual health tests.

Annual physical examinations are generally covered by health insurance or you can also get it for free or at a minimum cost. Routine tests are critically important to detect health problems at an early stage before they grow into a serious health issue.

15   Be kind to yourself.

Treat yourself every now and then. These can just be simple pampering such as getting your hair done at a posh salon, or scheduling a massage appointment. Break away from the demands and pressures of daily living and allow yourself to slow down, recharge and find temporary relief.

16   Stay motivated.

It can be difficult to stay on track to a health and fitness program if you are no longer motivated. Seek inspiration and find ways to stay motivated to make smarter choices and right decisions every single day. You are constantly faced with choices that pose real temptations such as choosing between watching TV and working out, or choosing between a chocolate chip cookie and a piece of fruit.

17   Drink alcohol in moderation.

Alcohol shows up in almost every social event, especially during the holiday season. Learn to limit your intake to no more than one or two drinks since too much alcohol can disrupt your sleep and make you feel sluggish the following day, not to mention contribute to extra calories.

18   Limit sugar in your diet as much as possible.

We all know how sugar can be detrimental to health. The problem is it is in so many products so make sure to read the labels and learn to steer clear from any processed food products as it is most likely laden with too much sugar. Nutrition experts recommend limiting added sugar to no more than 10 tablespoons a day.

However, sugar can come in so many forms and under many names. Be extra wary on food products that contain the following:

- Glucose
- High fructose corn syrup
- Lactose

- Honey
- Fruit juice concentrates
- Molasses
- Maltose
- Sucrose
- Brown sugar
- Fructose

To give you an idea on the sugar content on some of the popular food products and beverages, refer to the data provided below:

- Regular soda   33%
- Candies   16%
- Cakes, pies and cookies   13%
- Fruit drinks   10%

Individuals who are constantly exposed to consumption of food products with high sugar content also increase their calorie intake and lower micronutrient supply.

19   Eat complex carbohydrates.

When it comes to losing weight and eating right, we all know we need to watch our carb intake. However, there are good carb sources that are perfectly safe to eat such as whole grains. FDA recommends 55% of daily calorie supply should be derived from carbohydrates. However, you need to closely monitor the sources of your carbohydrates as there is a huge difference between complex and simple carbohydrates.

Simple carbohydrates are normally found in pasta, rice, white potatoes along with some daily products. They contain high amounts of sugar that need to be broken down by the body. While this type of sugar provides energy, when not consumed, it will be converted to fat. This is the reason why many diets restrict the intake of carbohydrate-rich food. Simple carbohydrates can contribute to weight gain and are especially risky for pregnant women.

On the other hand, complex carbohydrates, while containing sugar also feature more complex chains, making it more difficult to break it down. This allows the human body ample time to use it longer. Another great benefit of complex carbs is the high fiber content, which add bulk to the diet, effectively warding of hunger at the same time alleviate and prevent constipation.

20   Cut down your caffeine.

Too much caffeine can be bad for your health. Limit your intake to at least one to two cups per day. However, a lot of people are actually silent victims of caffeine addiction with common symptoms that include irritability, anxiety, upset stomach, poor concentration, insomnia, and depression, among others.

Caffeine has become a lifetime drug addiction for many. In essence, it is a toxic substance that should always be taken in moderation. Like sugar, it has the tendency to overstimulate and then weaken the adrenal glands, which results to fatigue. People suffering anxiety attacks and insomnia and are caffeine addicts will require high levels of tranquilizers to aid relaxation and promote better sleep.

If you are not really hooked into drinking coffee, avoid the addiction at all cost. Like illegal drugs, caffeine also has its own host of unpleasant symptoms during withdrawal.

21   Push yourself.

You have probably heard advices telling you not to be hard on yourself. There is a huge difference between castigating yourself and adhering to selfodisciplen. Push yourself in a positive way but don't allow self-imposed pressure overwhelm you instead of motivate you.

22   Take it from Nike, JUST DO IT.

Most times we find ourselves willing victims of procrastination, always putting of exercise and diet for another day. Instead of overthinking and over-planning things, just go ahead and do it. You will soon find your momentum and discover that one hardest part is getting started.

23   Watch what you put on your grocery cart.

One cardinal rule you need to vigilantly follow is to never do your grocery shopping on an empty stomach. Otherwise, you will find yourself falling prey to compulsive buying. Instead, prepare a list of things you need and but make sure to stick to that list. Make sure to stick to whole, fresh food products.

24   Take 5 to 6 meals a day.

Many people who go on a diet often complain about dealing with hunger pangs and that sense of deprivation. One way to combat this is to replace your 3 large meals with 5 to 6 small ones. This will not only prevent you from overeating and caving in to temptation, regular food intake can pump up your metabolism.

25 Eat at home.

One major contributing factor to weight gain is the propensity to eat fast food meals, takeout and microwave dinners – all of which are heavily laden with calories. While it may extra effort to prepare meals from scratch, you should never compromise your health with convenience. There are quick and no-fuss recipes online you can use to whip up meals in minutes.

26 Incorporate physical activities in your daily life.

Maximize every chance you get to move your body and work out. You don't really need to go to the gym to burn calories, there are so many ways you can pump up your metabolism by making simple changes, such as taking the stairs instead of the elevator, parking father away so you will be forced walk the rest of the way. Play with your kids and perform pushups during commercial breaks. Do everything you can to stay active all throughout the day.

27 Be selective on the shows you watch on TV.

The whole concept is to limit TV time before you unwittingly turn into a couch potato. If you tend to enjoy watching TV too much and too often, you won't realize how much time you spend in front of the boob tube.

According to studies, too much TV can lead to early death. Sedentary lifestyle can take off years from your life and increase the risk of heart disease. While TV in itself is not harmful, being in a constantly sitting position lead to the general absence of muscle movement, which can significantly disrupt the body's metabolism.

28 Make smart food choices.

Some diets impose impossible restrictions that are simply not practical and sustainable. You don't want to go on a diet on a specific period of time but cultivate a healthy living that will last a lifetime. This includes the small choices you make every single day.

29 Maintain at least one hobby.

Find an activity that you are passionate about that you probably won't mind doing for hours, may it be photography, vising museums or spending hours in a bookstore. Pursue things that bring the greatest joy.

30 Bask in love.

Whether you have a significant other, your family or friends, or even your pet dog, take time to connect and enjoy their company. Establish connections and nurture relationships. It can do wonders for your health and well-being.

31 Go organic.

You have probably heard reports on how even fresh produce today are exposed to chemicals and pesticides. It is generally best to get your food from organic sources. With the growing demand for such products, you can easily find different varieties and brands that are labeled organically grown or produced. However, be prepared to spend more for such products although, there is no price tag for good health, right?

32   Avoid negative people and situations.

Too much emotional stress can wreak havoc in your well-being. This does not mean you should avoid confrontations altogether, but learn to draw the lines. There is no use being around people who belittle you and undermine your dreams and goals. Prolonged exposure to stress can trigger binge eating and depression, which ultimately lead to weight gain.

33   Explore.

See the world or try out a sport. Move beyond your comfort zone every once in a while. It will do you good. Adding something new and pursuing something worthwhile will help keep you active and alive, as it breaks the usual humdrum. Open up to new experiences and be more accommodating to new changes. New experiences will lead to deeper self-discovery and more meaningful life.

34   Don't confuse thirst with hunger.

The human body has difficulty differentiating thirst from hunger. So when you are starting to feel hunger pangs, avoid indulging in food right away and instead drink a glass of water and check if you are still hungry.

35   Eat at a leisurely pace.

Enjoy your food and chew it thoroughly. It will usually take 20 minutes before you feel full so it's important not to gorge down your food, lest you overindulge.

A number of studies have confirmed that people who tend to eat slowly consume lesser amount of calories, enough to help you lose as much as 20 pounds per year. The brain takes time to register fullness of stomach, which means that by eating slowly, you have more time to realize you are already full.

36   Avoid stress eating.

A lot of people become unwitting victims to this pitfall. If you feel the need to binge, ask yourself what trigger it. It may be from feeling a sense of adequacy, agitation or depression. Properly identify and confront your emotions instead of taking out your frustration on food. It may help to write down what you feel or engage in activities that will distract you.

Awareness is key when combatting emotional or stress eating. This is because a lot of people actually tend to end more by simply not paying attention to what they put into their mouths. Eating without full awareness will lead to overeating, making poor food choices as well as the inability to truly enjoy food.

Whether you are working or lounging at the comfort of your home, avoid having food around areas that you can readily reach and eat mindlessly. Every time you feel urges and cravings, determine where it comes from. Practice restraint instead of succumbing to temptation.

37   Avoid eating while watching TV or going to the movies.

Many people don't realize how much food they consume while they are focused on their favorite movie or TV series. Avoid having food nearby or if you really need to snack, prepare something healthy like carrot sticks.

38   Teach yourself to control cravings.

One of the common downfalls of any diet programs is not the diet itself, but the individual's attitude towards food. Self-discipline is a very important trait you need to cultivate so you don't constantly cave in to temptation.

39   Get support from family and friends.

If you are following a special diet or a health regimen, let people who truly care about you know what you are into so they can understand and adjust accordingly. A support group is very important to help you start motivated and provide the affirmation and encouragement when you need it the most.

40   Beat temptations through distraction.

Every time you find it overly difficult to resist temptation, keep yourself busy so you don't have to dwell on the thought. Allowing yourself to be lured in indulging on one cookie will most likely lead to another one.

41   Keep a diary or journal.

It helps to write down your thoughts and feelings as it helps put things in perspective. It can also be a great way to track your progress if you are trying to lose weight.

42   Don't overlook the importance of emotional fitness.

Your emotional well-being is as important as your physical fitness. If you feel the need to vent or talk to sometime, seek the company of trusted friends or family. You can also consider taking therapy sessions.

43   Don't indulge too much on one thing.

Anything of excess can be a bad thing. Be smart on your choices and keep your food intake to a minimum. Eat to nourish and nurture the body and not become a glutton. Your overall well-being and health should always be given priority.

44   Find a fitness buddy.

If you are a people person, it may be easier to stick to a health and fitness program if you have someone who can share your journey. It is also more fun to engage in activities and try out healthy recipes with someone. You can also check out local organizations in your area.

45   Ride a bike to work.

If possible, you may want to consider riding a bicycle to work. It's a far healthier mode of transportation not to mention a cheaper alternative as well. If the distance between your home and work is no less than 8 kilometers, then you can consider taking a bicycle to work. However, before you do so make sure you take all the necessary precautions such as wearing a protective helmet and installing headlights.

46   Be conscious with your food portions.

Even if you are eating healthy, but you are eating too much of it, it defeats the purpose of diet and taking everything in moderation. Try not to eat meals that are no bigger that your first.

47   Increase fiber in your daily diet.

Fiber aids in weight loss and prevents constipation. It can also help avoid the buildup of toxins in the body, which may lead to other health complications.

Following a high-fiber diet can help effectively reduce the risks of heart diseases, colon cancer, diabetes as well as diverticular diseases. It also works well in lowering the cholesterol levels. To increase fiber in the diet, here are some basic guidelines:

•   Increase consumption of grains and cereals – oat bran, wheat germ, whole wheat flour products, high-fiber cereals and whole wheat crackers

•   Increase consumption of beans and legumes – kidney beans, legumes, and garbanzos

•   Fruits and veggies – fruits and vegetables, carrots, banana

48   Enjoy after dinner walks.

If you have your family around, establish the routine of enjoying quiet walks around the neighborhood. It's a great way to burn calories and bond.

According to studies, moderate intensity exercises like bricks walking can promote better weight loss. As a general rule, for you to shed of a single pound, you will need to burn about 3, 500 calories. A 30-minute walk helps to burn off an estimated 150 calories. Contrary to popular belief, walking after dinner will not cause muscle cramps.

49   Bake, steam or grill instead of frying.

Deep fried dishes are high in cholesterol, so it's best to avoid it. If you really need to use cooking oil in your meals, opt for olive oil as it is far healthier alternative.

50   Avoid eat all you can buffets.

You generally don't want to put yourself in a position where it is difficult to resist temptation.

51   Only take enough food you can eat.

Avoid indulging in second and third helpings. Only place enough food on your plate that you are willing to consume, so you can avoid over-indulging.

It can also be a good idea to only get enough food from the pan and leave the rest. This way, you will only consume the food available on the table and avoid excessive eating. If you plan to make large dishes to store, store it in containers and freeze. This provides you convenient food alternative then you travel or for office lunches.

52   Start your meals with salads.

Before enjoying the main course, have a plate of green salad although you need to pay attention on the choice of dressing. This will help you feel fuller as soon as you are ready to start with the main course.

By filling up your body with water-rich and fiberorich food, you can effectively avoid overindulging on high calorie meals. In fact, in a study conducted at Penn State, eating salads first can reduce consumption of calories by as much as 12%.

53   Replace sugar with honey.

Consider using organic honey instead of sugar in your beverages and baked products as a healthier option. If you should use table sugar, opt for the brown one as it contains lesser chemicals.

If you are trying to cut down on sugar consumption, honey presents a perfect alternative since honey is generally sweeter than regular table sugar, which means you need to only use lesser amount. However, be extra careful when substituting sweeteners in recipe since honey has its own distinct flavor, which can potentially ruin your baked goodies.

54   Avoid skipping meals.

A lot of people seem to think that the best way to lose weight is to skip meals. This can actually have a detrimental effect as it causes fluctuations on the blood sugar levels and trigger excessive hunger which can lead to overeating. Stick to eating small, frequent meals.

55   Trade baked goodies with fresh fruits.

Pastries, cakes and cookies are all high in carbohydrates and sugar which can lead to weight gain. Have a piece of apple instead or any other fruit in season.

56   When eating out, choose the healthiest meals.

Learn the art of choosing healthier meal options. It can also help if you share your meals with the people you are with if it is an informal gathering.

57   Avoid using condiments.

Some condiments are generally bad for the health so try to avoid using them as much as possible. While condiments are known to add more flavor and aroma in food, there are those that come fully loaded with sugar which poses serious health risks. Here are some pointers on what you can use and what to avoid:

Enjoy the following condiments:
- Mustard
- Hot sauce
- Vinegars
- Cream cheese
- Worcestershire sauce
- Horseradish
- Pesto
- Soy sauce
- Sour cream

Avoid the following condiments:
- Barbecue sauce

- Maple syrup
- Teriyaki sauce
- Ketchup
- Cocktail sauce
- Regular jellies and jams

58 When travelling, check out gym facilities.

Travelling out of town or out of the country should not disrupt you regular exercise regimen. Check out available facilities and include exercise in your itinerary. You can also bring along a few simple gym equipment like skipping rope or an elastic band if you want to exercise at the comforts of your hotel room.

59 Do your research on local restaurants that offer healthy alternatives.

When being in an unfamiliar place it can be all too easy to eat what is convenient and readily available. To help you stick to your diet, check out healthy options within the area. You can always ask in front desk for assistance.

60 Bring your lunch.

Instead of grabbing a quick bite at the cafeteria or a nearby fast food chain, bring along your lunch by storing it in a brown bag. This will give you better control on what type of food you eat and how much you consume. It can be good idea to prepare large batches of meals so you can bring along extras for your lunch.

61   Trade your recliner with an exercise ball.

The growing trend among modern offices today is the use of exercise balls in place of ordinary office chairs. This is a perfect option for people whose work requires them to spend long hours behind the desk. Exercise balls will require you to maintain proper posture and use muscles for balance. It is a good passive workout for desk bound employees.

62   Use your break time wisely.

Instead of taking a nap or chatting with your colleagues, maximize your break time by going out for a short walk. It can be good idea to bring along some comfy shoes that you can use.

63   Conduct a meeting on the go.

Instead of staying cooped up in the conference room, maximize time by conducting your meeting outdoors or while walking towards another location. This will not only save you time, it presents a perfect excuse to stretch your legs and exercise.

64   Invest in a pedometer.

This is a small device you can wear to measure the number of steps you make in a day. This will help you keep track and serve as a reminder all throughout the day. It can also be a great tool to you reach your fitness objectives even while at the office or while running some errands.

65 Learn to modify.

Every so often you may find yourself in situations where it is difficult to stick to your fitness routine. The trick here is to learn to adjust to situations. If you don't have dumbbells around you can use canned goods or water bottles as alternative options. Learn to make use of available resources and be creative.

66 Take vacations from work, not from good health.

Travelling and enjoying a holiday vacation should not be an excuse to indulge in foods that are generally bad for your health. Stick to your healthy food regimen.

67 Learn to express your feelings.

Keeping your emotions bottled up, you contribute to stress and increases the risks of health related problems such as heart attacks, substance abuse, depression and excessing stress. Define the underlying negative emotions and determine its triggers. Everything is a matter of perspective. Learn to embrace positivity in your words, actions and thoughts.

68 Maintain a positive attitude.

Life will not always go your way. Instead of wallowing in failures and disappointments, learn to brush it off and move forward. Whether it is a failed relationship, a lost opportunity or an unsavory situation, choose to see the positive side of things and maintain a happy disposition. This will help you channel your energies to the right direction and rise up to the challenges.

69 Try meditation.

This involves control of breathing patterns and enhancing focus. This will help you clear away mental cobwebs and maintain better perspective on situations. By learning the right breathing patterns, you will be able to provide your brain the right oxygen supply to clear away mental disturbances.

70 Reinforce your faith.

Develop and seek spiritual enlightenment and focus beyond material wealth. This will help you attain lasting happiness and satisfaction which are difficult to derive from material possessions. By reinforcing your faith, you can also promote better overall health and well-being.

71 Stay young at heart.

Don't take everything too seriously. Learn to enjoy life's simple pleasures. Laughter is the best anti-aging solution available for free. It can also help boost the immune system.

72 Stay in touch with friends.

Despite the popularity of online social networking sites, it should not replace your personal interactions with people around you. Indulge in regular conversations and preserve real life social networks by joining groups and staying in touch with friends or planning activities together.

73   Perform regular stretching exercises.

Stretching is the best way to work out a few kinks and aches from staying in a position for far too long, like working in a computer. Check out some great stretching exercises readily available online and discover how simple stretches can aid in relaxations and ease muscle tension.

74   Keep talking.

According to research, talking at least ten minutes a day to another person can promote better brain function and enhance memory. Brief chats can actually boost brain power compared to watching TV. Another study also revealed that social people have longer life span.

75   Stop smoking.

One can't stress enough the risks and ill-effects of smoking. It limits the oxygen supply of the body and result to a host of health complications including shortened life expectancy rate. It has also been found that smoking can indirectly contribute to back pain.
Smoking also has adverse effects on people around you. Second hand smokers have been known to suffer significant increased risks of health complications that can even lead to death.

76   Aim high.

Set your weight and health goals and break it into small milestones. This will keep you motivated and focused on achieving your goals. Write it down and place it in places where you can regularly read it, serving as a constant reminder. Post a copy on your refrigerator, work desk and laptop.

77   Keep yourself updated.

Conduct regular research and stay updated on the latest health discoveries and equip yourself with the knowledge to make smart food choices. The Internet provides a plethora of resources on new exercise routines, new health spas in your area, and any other health and fitness-related interests.

78   Know your body.

Determine what are factors that trigger weight gain and learn what are the best nutrition for your specific body type. This will help you in making day to day decisions. There are different types of body, which will require different weight loss and nutrition approaches. Take time to study each one and determine which particular body type or combination of body type you actually have.

79   Go easy on the barbie.

Compared to other dishes and food preparations, barbeques are not hygienic and may increase the risks of stomach and intestine problems and infections.

80   Treat your brain like any other muscle.

Much like any other muscle in the body, your brain also needs regular exercise. Enjoy board games, crossword puzzles and any other activity that presents mental challenge.

81 Get nutty.

Nuts are healthy snack options, which can effectively stave off food cravings. Make sure to choose the unsalted and roasted varieties as they are known to be free from sugars and sodium.

82 Stay protected.

Don't forget to apply sunblock, especially during hot, humid days. Protect your skin from sun damage, which can lead to premature aging. If possible wear protective headgear when exposed to direct sunlight. Excessive exposure to harmful sun's rays can cause cancer and wrinkles.

83 Mind your posture.

Protect your back from unnecessary damage due to poor posture. Maintaining proper posture can enhance mental focus and promote better blood circulation.

84 Avoid processed food products.

Always choose fresh, whole foods as much as possible. In general, foods that are packaged in boxes, bags and cans have been altered and are highly processed, which makes them devoid from essential nutrients and instead laden with preservations and chemicals.

85 Always carry a water bottle wherever you go.

This is one of the most practical ways you can stay fit and hydrated all throughout the day. This can effectively reduce hunger cravings, prevent you from overeating, prevent irritability, headaches and cramps and promote proper body functioning.

86 Get plenty of fresh air.

Revitalize your body by inhaling fresh air. Go outside and take deep breaths. Enclosed work spaces can reduce natural air flow, which makes you more susceptible to diseases. Enjoy walks with your dog, if you have one.

87 Take advantage for natural sunlight.

Early morning sunlight can help boost immune system and has been known to combat depression.

88 Take the stairs.

Instead of using the elevator, use the opportunity for some quick workout by taking the stairs.

89   For women, visit gynecologist regularly.

Females 18 and above should undergo annual physical examination include Pap Smear test. In addition, those in their 40s should have mammograms along with regular breast self-examination to ensure early detection.

90   Walk and stretch during road travel.

When taking road trips, make sure to take frequent stops so you have a chance to walk around the vicinity and stretch the muscles. This will not only protect your back and help you burn calories, stretching can also help you start more alert on the road when driving. Regular stops will help you feel better upon reaching your destination.

91   Visit your dentist regularly.

Good oral hygiene is also an important part of overall health and wellness.

92   Workout with kids.

Spend the weekend with playing with kids. This is the perfect opportunity to bond and spend leisure time away from the daily stresses. Plan a park or beach outing or even a trip to the zoo. Keeping up with active toddlers and preschoolers can turn out to be a fun exercise for you.

93   Substitute emails for walks.

When working in an office, instead of emailing your colleague, grab this opportunity to walk over and discuss things personally instead of confining communication via email. This will not only speed up the communication process, it also provides you opportunities to stretch and walk.

94   Warm up before exercise.

Launching your body into an intense physical exercise with cold muscles can increase the risks of injuries. In fact, a lot of sports-related injuries can be prevented through proper stretching and warm ups. Whether it's a high impact sport like basketball, or a grueling game of golf, never undermine the importance of properly warming up the muscles to prevent strains and sprains as well as cramps.

95   Take a stand.

You will be surprised to know that standing can burn up to 34 more calories compared to sitting down. So you can ditch the standard work desk with one that features vertical adjustments. When answering phones, stand and walk around, so you can burn calories at the same time.

96   Park farther.

Instead of fighting over who gets the prime parking lot spot, choose to park farther, preferably a full block away from the office. This will give you the opportunity to walk and stretch on a daily basis.

97   Use chicken breast and take off the skin.

When cooking, work with breast portions as it contains the most amount of white meat. Since chicken meat is so versatile, you can use it in almost any type of preparation and dish. It's the perfect source of protein especially for people on a diet.

98   Learn to decipher food labels.

This is one skill that will prove handy when making smarter food choices. Learn to interpret and properly determine if it's a safe option or an unhealthy substitute.

99   Just chew it.

If you are dealing with sweet tooth, try substituting your usual dessert with gum. This will keep your mouth busy and provide distraction you need to keep your mind off dessert. However, you need to be extra careful when dealing with sugar-free varieties. A lot of people actually have hypersensitivity to sugar substitutes such as sucralose and sorbitol. In fact, these sugar substitutes have been link to a number of gastrointestinal problems, such as bloating, diarrhea, constipation and cramping, among others. If you don't want to take your chance on sugar-free varieties, you will be happy to known that stick of regular gum contains about 5 to 10 calories.

100 Always choose to plan ahead.

It can be significantly easier to stick to eating regimen if you plan ahead. Prepare the menu for the following week so you don't have to spend extra time racking your brain on what to cook and how to prepare your food. Having a weekly menu can also effectively discourage the need to order food delivery and take outs.

101   Search for healthy alternatives. With more and more people seeking healthier options, a lot of traditional dishes today are available in healthier versions. For example, you can replace regular pasta noodles with squash spaghetti. It can be fun to explore your options so constantly research online. By learning ways to provide healthier alternatives, you won't feel overly deprived when undergoing a restrictive diet.

101 Keep moving forward.

People tend to be more motivated when they have an aim. They normally only react when they want an end result. So the lesson here is to always have a goal, and not just with your health and fitness but your overall wellbeing.

Conclusion

Up until today, it is very much a struggle and constant battle on the survival of the fittest. By keeping a healthy body and eating right, you open yourself up to a great new world of opportunities.

As the saying goes, if you want to be successful, you have to act, feel and look every bit as successful as you want to be. These days, financial status is not the only yardstick used to measure success. Appearance of a healthy and fit body is also critically important in wielding respect and commanding authority.

Incorporate all these tips, tricks and pointers into your lifestyle. While it may take a while to adjust and transition into a number of changes, investing in good health will never be too expensive.